Outliving

Average

Living longer in physical and emotional

health

Velma S. Haveman

Disclaimer

Table of Contents

Introduction

The average longevity has expanded by roughly 25 years throughout the previous century. At the same time, we've raised the burden of sickness. Despite living longer, we are not growing healthier. The bulk of chronic diseases and cancers attack at a later age, with the extra 25 years of life that modern medicine has provided us. Is it a wise compromise?

While performing a research, Perls noticed that many persons had reservations about surviving a long life, which impeded them from recognizing the significance of keeping healthy behaviors. Some persons feel that as you age, your health deteriorates, and they wouldn't want to live to that age. That argument is actually terribly flawed, he says.

Age-related changes influence many parts of life, including the physical, mental, social, emotional, and sexual. You may perceive some of these changes as good and others as undesirable. It could be challenging to reconcile proactive actions to safeguard your health with maximizing the beneficial qualities of aging.

Whether we are young or old, longevity is an issue that concerns us all. This suggests that if you want to live a long and healthy life, you should start making arrangements for it as early as possible, as this book explains.
 health with maximizing the beneficial qualities of aging.
Whether we are young or old, longevity is an issue that concerns us all. This suggests that if you want to live a long and healthy life, you should start making arrangements for it as early as possible, as this book explains.

CHAPTER ONE

Concepts of longevity, healthspan, and life expectancy

Longevity is the capacity to endure sufficiently beyond the usual death age for a species. One may conceive of longevity as the average lifetime under optimal circumstances. The expected lifespan of a person relies on their birth year, present age, and a range of demographic parameters, such as their gender. It is commonly characterized statistically as the normal number of years left in one's life at a certain age. Thus, life expectancy simply shows the average longevity of the population. The maximum lifetime, on the other hand, specifies how long it has been observed that members of a group would live between conception and death. The word "health span" defines the length of time in a person's life when they are in exceptional health. As a result, a person may become unwell early in life and nonetheless survive for a number of years. The health span is consequently shorter or, at most, equal to the lifetime. Life expectancy is the amount of time between conception and death that at least one person in a population may anticipate surviving. We may wish to live a long life in order to travel widely and spend a lot of time with our loved ones. However, living a long life does not mean that one will do so in good health if they are constrained by a sickness or handicap. The number of persons over 65 has increased faster than that of other age groups as a consequence of rising life expectancies and lower birth rates. Even yet, more years are being wasted in bad health. Longevity comprises two components. The first item to take into consideration is your actual longevity, but a second component that is as significant is your quality of life, generally referred to as your health span. The second element in our goal to live a long life is to maintain and develop both our mental and physical performance.

We will look at a person's lifetime as well as their health span in order to encourage longer, healthier years of living. Your present actions could affect how long you remain healthy or how you grow in the future. There is never a poor time to start, even though it is best to get started as soon as practical. Centenarians aren't as uncommon as they used to be. In the UK, there were 15,120 centenarians alive in 2020, roughly double the number from 2002, according to the Office for National Statistics.

What Age-Related Processes Are Normal and What Aren't?

To maintain your health, you must first be conscious of the
mental and physical changes that aging typically brings about. The following are some of the most frequent physiological changes you may see:

- **The Bones:** Our bones lose density or mass as we age, which contributes to osteoporosis and makes them thinner and more fragile. Your chance of breaking bones, especially spinal fractures, which may diminish your height and cause you to slouch, increases if you have low bone mass. Males may also have osteoporosis and reduced bone density, but women are more prone to these diseases. Be sure to go over your osteoporosis preventative alternatives with your doctor. Often, the first thing you notice is a fractured bone.

- **The Heart:** Blood pressure rises as a consequence of arteriosclerosis, a disorder that causes big arteries to harden with age. In addition, plaque commonly accumulates on the arterial walls, hardening and narrowing the arteries and limiting blood flow to the heart. The formation of fatty deposits is known as atherosclerosis, and the buildup of plaque in the arteries that carry blood to the heart is known as coronary artery disease. Both illnesses are important risk factors for heart attacks. Even if not all of the heart and blood vessel alterations brought on by age can be averted, a balanced diet and regular exercise may nearly always help to maintain your arteries and heart healthy for longer.

- **The Mind:** The Centers for Disease Control and Prevention (CDC) indicate that mild forgetfulness is a frequent aging symptom. Additionally, individuals might have a difficult time multitasking or digesting new information. If memory loss and confusion linger longer than the odd "senior moment," it's not normal, and you should visit a doctor. You might be in the early stages of dementia, but you could potentially have a curable brain illness.
- **The inner digestive system:** Aging causes your digestive system to slow

down and not contract as frequently as it did when you were younger, which may contribute to constipation, stomach discomfort, and nausea. Many drugs produce constipation as a harmful effect. In order to avoid these digestive disorders, the Mayo Clinic suggests eating a diet high in fiber, drinking enough water, staying as active as you can, and striving to manage your stress.

- **The Senses:** Your five senses—hearing, vision, taste, smell, and touch—might not be as keen as they once were, according to Medline Plus. Due to structural changes in the ear, you might have some hearing loss, which could also influence your balance. You might need reading glasses if your eyesight begins to degrade. You might start to lose your sense of taste as your body's supply of taste buds drops. Tastes may not appear as distinct or vivid to you as a result. Your sense of smell may weaken as you age because of reduced mucus production and a loss of nerve endings in the nose. You might also be less sensitive to touch, discomfort, pressure, and vibration, but some individuals find their sensitivity to touch increases with skin thinning.

- **The gums and teeth:** Your teeth's protective hard enamel may begin to disintegrate as you grow older, increasing your chance of acquiring cavities. Additionally, as you age, the nerves in your teeth may shrink, making you less sensitive to pain and maybe delaying the finding of cavities or fissures in the tooth's outer layer, according to the American Dental Association (ADA). A research published in the American Journal of Public Health in June 2017 indicated that moderate to severe gum disease affects more than half of people over the age of 65. According to the same research, 400 regularly used drugs may induce dry mouth, which enhances the risk of dental issues.

- **The Skin:** As you age older, your skin loses elasticity and may start to droop and wrinkle. However, the more you guard your skin from smoking and the sun when you are younger, the better it will appear as you age. The American Academy of Dermatology suggests sunscreen and moisturizer as the two most crucial anti-aging products you should be utilizing. If you wear a hat with a brim, the skin on your scalp and face will also be covered. To stop more aging and minimize your chance of skin cancer, protect your skin as soon as you can.
- **Your Sexual Function:** When menstruation ends and hormone levels decline during menopause, many women suffer physical changes, including less vaginal lubrication. The North American

Menopause Society notes that these changes might also make you less interested in having sex. According to the American Sexual Health Association, erectile dysfunction is a regular side effect of aging for men, however, it is not a natural aspect of getting older and could be an indication of another condition or a drug's harmful effects. Thankfully, a lot of these physical abnormalities may be swiftly addressed or, in the case that they cannot, could be endured by willing partners who are open to trying new things.

You don't have to allow these physiological changes to keep you down, even though many of them are inescapable as we age. You may do a variety of other things to safeguard your body and maintain it in the best possible shape. Understanding what is typical for your body as it ages and what is not is vital. Aging need not always be associated with a variety of medical difficulties or a bad quality of life.

Warning Signs to Watch Out For

It's tempting to blame exhaustion or a poor attitude to growing older, but this isn't always the case. It is not natural to feel fatigued or unsatisfied all the time, regardless of your age. If you feel less compelled or driven to participate in activities you used to appreciate, arrange an appointment with your doctor. You might be suffering from depression or another ailment that needs to be addressed right now. What additional warning indicators should you look out for? Any of the following symptoms should be investigated by a doctor since they could signal a significant health problem:

- unexpected weakness or tiredness
- breathing difficulties
- sensation of chest pressure

- Loss of coordination or balance, particularly on one side of your body, numbness or tingling
- difficulties swallowing or speaking profuse perspiration
- sudden eyesight loss or blurriness
- There is obvious swelling even if you haven't recently been wounded.
- rapid weight loss
- persistent bewilderment
- Bruises that never seem to heal

With early medical intervention, many individuals may overcome major physical difficulties and even flourish later if they take the chance to strengthen their concentration on living healthy and meaningful lives.

Myths about aging you shouldn't believe
It's vital to eradicate the various age-related beliefs in order to age successfully. Instead of just diminishing, the aging brain enjoys a

number of neurochemical advantages. Now let's look at two additional age-related fallacies that need to be refuted.

The first misconception is regarding memory loss. How often have you heard that memory loss comes with being older? Contrary to what many people assume, memory function is significantly more complex. One example is that, in line with studies, individuals of all ages may have difficulty with short-term memory. Simply mentioned, when we're young, we choose to reject it by stating that we're sleepy, overworked, or even simply having a lousy day. However, older adults who experience short-term memory loss are more prone to feel that it is a marker of cognitive decline.

Additionally, older brains fare better in terms of memory. This applies to our capacity to form judgments and conclusions based on patterns. When presented with difficult circumstances,

older brains are better equipped to remember earlier experiences and the neural connections their brains built over those encounters.
Due to their expanded memory capacity, older brains are better at zooming out and acquiring a bird's eye perspective of things. As a result, older individuals are better at making decisions, particularly when presented with ethically complicated options like whether to continue in a relationship or not or whether confronting your boss is the correct course of action. If your issue demands impartiality and intellect, seek elderly adults for assistance—their minds are genuinely better suited to it!

Another misconception is that if an older person takes up a new talent or interest, they are past their prime and won't be able to do as much as they did when they were younger. This is untrue, to put it simply. Take a peek at Anna Mary Robertson's artworks shown in the Smithsonian and the Met Museum of Art in

New York. Robertson didn't start painting until she was 75 years old. KFC's founder Harland Sanders is yet another fantastic instance in point. He spent his entire life jumping between several occupations before launching KFC at the age of 62. After fourteen years, he sold it for the equivalent of $32 million.

Aging is not generally accompanied by bad health. In addition to having a long lifetime, persons who survive to reach 100 years old may escape significant sickness until later in life. Even if diabetes, dementia, and heart disease all have increasing risks with age, it is still possible to live a long, healthy life free of diseases.

CHAPTER TWO

In the era of chronic illnesses, medical practice needs to be reevaluated

A chronic illness is a sickness or condition that affects human health and is lasting or has other long-term impacts. The word "chronic" is typically used to describe symptoms that linger for more than three months.

Chronic illnesses are now the major cause of adult mortality in practically every country, and over the next 10 years, that number is anticipated to climb by another 17%. A third of individuals on the earth suffer from various chronic ailments. In the US, four out of ten persons and six out of ten have three or more chronic diseases. According to projections, chronic illnesses would be the cause of 35 million of the 58 million fatalities that will occur in 2005. The World Health Organization maintains that since chronic illnesses cannot be spread from one person to another, they are not communicable. They develop slowly and persist for a very long duration.

Leading chronic illnesses are largely brought on by unhealthy behaviors like smoking, inactivity, bad eating habits, and binge drinking. The most frequent chronic diseases in affluent nations include arthritis, cardiovascular disorders including heart attacks and stroke, malignancies such as breast and colon cancer, diabetes, epilepsy, and seizures, obesity, and issues with the mouth. Elderly individuals are influenced by each of these disorders. A scenario where chronic illnesses (CDs) are on the increase is exceedingly harmful for the general public's health as well as the affected communities and economy. Chronic illnesses' effects and profiles have frequently not been completely acknowledged until recently. In general, chronic illnesses cannot be treated by medicine, avoided by vaccination, or healed on their own.

Characteristics of Chronic Disease

Most chronic conditions are defined by:

- difficult explanations numerous hazards
- Long latency periods (the span of time between the development of a disease and the manifestation of symptoms)
- chronic illness functional incapacity or constraint.

Many chronic diseases are not totally cured, and most do not go away on their own. Some of diseases, including heart disease and stroke, can be deadly immediately away. Others, such as diabetes, require frequent care over time. Most chronic diseases, like arthritis, continue for the entire of a person's life but do not necessarily cause death.

Common Chronic Conditions

Although many diseases may be labeled as chronic, there are 13 main chronic ailments that cause a considerable burden in terms of morbidity, mortality, and healthcare costs: Type 2 diabetes, osteoporosis, asthma, chronic obstructive pulmonary disease (COPD), chronic renal disease, oral disease, colorectal cancer, lung cancer, cardiovascular disease, stroke, and other disorders. People with chronic diseases need to manage their therapies, make sure they are aware about their condition and treatment choices, keep their emotions in control so they can tolerate unpleasant feelings, and retain their confidence and good self-image.

Chronic Disease Management and Interventions

Improved chronic illness treatment and prevention demand major investment. Giving patients who need it access to palliative care is an essential step in the diagnosis, screening, and treatment of chronic illnesses. To encourage early identification and speedy treatment of chronic illnesses while delivering high-impact medicines, a primary healthcare strategy may be employed.

There is emerging evidence that diet has a considerable influence on the development and treatment of chronic illnesses. A strategy to lessen patient suffering and the financial burden that chronic diseases impose on the healthcare system is dietary recommendations. As a consequence, dietitians need to be contacted for nutrition-related guidance, particularly in situations of chronic illnesses that are connected to food. The study implies that these medicines are worthwhile financial investments because, if administered to patients in a timely way, they may obviate the need for more costly therapy. It appears doubtful that nations with insufficient health insurance would offer everyone access to important chronic illness medicines.

Both the worldwide aim of a 25% relative decline in the risk of premature mortality from chronic diseases by 2025 and the Sustainable Development Goals (SDGs) target of a third reduction in premature deaths from CDs by 2030 depend on the management of chronic disease treatments. The WHO proposes three guiding principles in their article titled "Integrating the response to mental disorders and other chronic diseases in health care systems" for an integrated strategy for treating these conditions:

There needs to be a genuine public health strategy. In addition to the provision of readily accessible, all-inclusive services that are coordinated to fit the requirements of individuals who have been identified, this necessitates putting an emphasis on the promotion of wellness and avoidance of disease throughout life.

The delivery of health services or technical improvements is only one component of a systems approach, which also needs good administration, proper financing, and timely information.
A comprehensive, cross-cutting government strategy is necessary. In order to address the physical, social, and financial ramifications of mental disorders and other chronic conditions, the health sector cannot or should not act alone.

Physiotherapy and Chronic Disease
Physical therapists concentrate on both the treatment and prevention of chronic ailments. Just a fraction of the jobs they fulfill are as follows:

- Exercise and education seminars for patients with chronic conditions are also arranged, in addition to prescribing and carrying out therapeutic exercise programs for individuals or groups.

- Asthma patients are treated with cardio-pulmonary rehabilitation and recommended exercise routines.
- Diabetics and those at risk for the illness are offered exercise treatment to help them regulate their blood sugar levels.
- programs for persons with different heart diseases as well as cardiac rehabilitation.

There are therapies available to lower the risk of osteoporotic fracture, such as therapeutic exercise. Health promotion and education that takes place in a number of contexts, such as one-on-one counseling, organized group sessions, disease-specific self-management seminars, and information on lifestyle changes including quitting smoking, drinking less alcohol, managing pain and exhaustion, etc.

In practically every nation, chronic illnesses are already the primary cause of mortality, and the danger to people's lives, health, and the growth of their countries' economies is expanding quickly. The information is at hand to avert this menace and save millions of lives. Many nations have proved the value of cost and effective initiatives and the know-how necessary to execute them. Combining current therapies as part of a holistic, integrated strategy may assist the world in accomplishing its objective of avoiding chronic illnesses.

CHAPTER THREE

Living longer by eating less

Cutting calories helps individuals live longer and age more slowly. A stringent low-calorie diet may also reduce or halt aging in monkeys, according to ongoing studies. Lower daily calorie intake has been reported to promote lifespan in yeast and mice. But the mechanism underlying the benefits has confounded academics for years.

The first genetic indication for how eating less might lengthen life has recently been uncovered, according to research. It appears in Science's edition of September 22. According to Massachusetts Institute of Technology molecular scientist Leonard Guarente, yeast cells may survive 25% longer if their glucose intake is lowered by as much as 75%.

What does it mean to enhance your nutrition, and how do you go about doing so?
Keeping poor meals to a minimum is a fantastic place to start. There are appropriate portion reductions for ice cream, salt, and French fries. But it's not simply what you consume, according to this recent research and a lot of professional advice. Furthermore, what you consume matters. It's also vital to consume more nutrient-dense meals.

Data on food availability, patient surveys from 1990 to 2012, facts on cardiovascular mortality in 2015, and statistics on food availability were contributed for this study by the Food and Agriculture Organization of the United Nations. They determined that inadequate consumption of whole grains, nuts, seeds, and seeds, as well as trans fat—a particularly unhealthy form of unsaturated fat frequently found in processed foods as "partially hydrogenated oils"—were the primary causes of the early cardiovascular deaths of more than 220,000 men and roughly 190,000 women.

The advice to adopt a nutritious diet in order to be as healthy as possible has been heard by everyone. Changing your diet could have a major influence, even if it's easier said than done. This is accurate, according to a recent research that investigated the influence of dietary adjustments on cardiovascular mortality in this nation. The choice? A boost in nutrition may avert more than 400,000 fatalities every year.

Here's a brief reminder that reducing calories is not the same as starving. Starvation arises when someone deprives himself of food and nutrition. Contrarily, calorie restriction implies regulated eating (by limiting the overall amount of calories ingested) without resulting in malnutrition. When we speak about calorie restriction for life, it's not simply about foregoing soft drinks and dessert. It implies a large decrease in daily calorie consumption.

Yale University researchers believe that cutting down on calories helps "rejuvenate" a vital component of your immune system. Adults who lowered their calorie intake by roughly 14% performed better in their thymus glands. This is roughly comparable to 300 calories for males who stick to the 2,500 calorie intake for men and 2,000 calorie advice for women each day. Inflammation, which arises when the immune system overreacts and leads to a multitude of disorders, may be averted by calorie restriction, according to experts.

How may calorie restriction help us live longer?
The obvious remedy is to modify metabolic health. Reduced food intake indicates that the body has less food to digest. Additionally, since eating less leads to a net weight reduction when

you restrict calories, your body requires less energy to sustain the reduced body mass, which slows your metabolic rate.

Caloric restriction reduces blood sugar levels and may boost ketone levels while maintaining them within acceptable limits if done effectively (i.e., by paying attention to the amount and quality of calories taken). When we are in a calorie deficit, our bodies start turning to their fat stores for energy. When these fats are turned into energy (a process known as beta-oxidation), molecules known as ketones are created and start to appear in the blood and urine. When we switch from consuming glucose to using ketones as fuel, our metabolic balance improves.

Caloric restriction has so far proven extraordinary advantages for health in a broad variety of animals, including:

- decreased vulnerability to seizures in epileptic mice

- improved chicken production and fertility
  Animals with delayed development of
  age-related diabetes had reduced levels of
  oxidative stress, which is wonderful for
  lifespan.
- increased longevity and health

The advantages of calorie restriction for healthier and longer lives have been established in various studies on single-cell organisms and animals, but in-depth study on people is still absent.

These data suggest that there are major health advantages, which is a terrific signal that we are on the right route. Calorie restriction appears to be advantageous for our cardiovascular health, which is vital for our lifespan.

The best course of action may not, however, be to merely cut down on your food intake. It is crucial to make sure your dietary demands are addressed. The greatest method to begin your road toward longevity by focusing on your food habits is to chat with a doctor. The quality of the food you eat, not the volume, is ultimately what matters most for your health.

Does a healthy Diet Prolong Life?

Healthy eating may help you live longer at any age! According to an intriguing modeling study by a group of researchers from Norway that was just published in PLOS Medicine, raising your daily intake of vegetables, legumes, whole grains, and nuts while lowering your consumption of processed meat and sugar-sweetened beverages is predicted to increase life expectancy.

The researchers' "optimal" healthy diet was defined as being heavy in processed foods, sweets, and red meat. If you shift from this diet to this one at the age of 20, you may add more than 10 years to your life expectancy. If giving up junk food altogether sounds impossible, there is good news: the researchers showed that eating fewer processed foods while still consuming them in some capacity (what they labeled a "feasible" healthy diet) may nevertheless increase a 20-year-old's longevity by roughly 7 years. What about people who are older than middle age and have a significant history of consuming junk food? According to the model, moving to a practical and nutritious diet at the age of 60 may result in a 5 or 9-year boost in life expectancy.

How may a good diet prolong your life?
"You are what you eat," a statement that is well-known to most people, but what does it truly mean? It is ridiculous to suppose that what is put into your body doesn't actually affect who you are. And that includes your predisposition for living longer...or dying sooner.
Most of the body's cells are short-lived and frequently need to be replaced. (Your skin cells are replaced every four to six weeks, while stomach epithelial cells normally only survive approximately five days.) Think of your body as

a factory that makes new cells; it is your obligation to make sure that it receives the finest raw materials (nutrients) essential to build new, healthy cells.

Fruits, vegetables, legumes, and other healthy meals give fantastic building blocks, but over time, you won't profit from the very tasty, high-sugar items that may pull you in. Beyond that, good food delivers a range of additional advantages, including a lower risk of heart disease and other chronic illnesses associated with nutrition, improved blood pressure, a stronger immune system, and more. Undoubtedly, a healthier diet makes it simpler to maintain a healthy weight.

Foods that may help you live longer
Diet and lifespan are issues that can never be completely understood. We do, however, at least have a fair understanding of which dietary categories may be able to predict success with longevity based on the information already

accessible. To live longer, regularly include these products in your menu:

- Vegetables: cruciferous vegetables like broccoli, cabbage, and kale as well as leafy greens, carrots, sweet potatoes, and leafy greens
- Brown rice, quinoa, buckwheat, oatmeal, and other whole grains
- Legumes: includes foods like pinto beans, chickpeas, almonds, soybeans, lentils, and peanuts. These plant-based meals are an excellent source of protein and fiber.
- The white meats: Salmon, chicken, turkey, and mahi-mahi
- Fruits: Avocados, apples, pomegranates, and berries strong in antioxidants like blueberries and strawberries are also wonderful selections.

Limit or stay away from certain meals

It is a dreadful fact that folks who hold the notion that "Life is too short to not eat dessert" may be producing a self-fulfilling prophecy. Regularly consuming a lot of fast food, sugary foods, and other items from the list below (along with other lifestyle choices) may actually lower longevity, in large part because these foods are associated with heart disease, the number one killer in the US. Therefore, it's necessary to fight the impulse to overindulge in harmful meals and create the habit of picking foods that progress rather than jeopardize your health.

Naturally, it's okay to reward yourself once in a while, but sticking to just these meals might wind up costing you:

- **Ultra-processed foods** are among the unhealthiest as they generally contain substantial quantities of added sugar, salt, oil, and harmful fats. Examples include soft beverages, packaged snacks, frozen meals, cereals, and ice cream. Ultra-processed meals are typically classified as "industrial products" because they are usually so changed that they comprise little to no whole, intact components. Surprisingly, ultra-processed foods account for more than 60% of the dietary energy ingested in the US. In a meta-analysis of observational studies, which looked at over 183,500 participants followed for a length ranging from 3.5 to 19 years, it was demonstrated that the greatest consumption of ultra-processed foods was related to an elevated risk of depression, cardiovascular disease, and all-cause mortality.

- **Meals cooked at a high temperature** It's not just the elements of a meal that matter; particular cooking techniques may change an otherwise nutritious dinner into something harmful. This is because boiling food at excessively high temperatures may generate harmful substances, most notably advanced glycation end products (AGEs), which are formed when glucose molecules attach to proteins and cause other proteins to cross-link. A greater risk of getting numerous chronic illnesses and early aging are both connected with AGEs. High-heat cooking techniques including frying, grilling, broiling, baking, and searing are to be avoided. The odd meal produced using these ways is okay, but aim to boil, steam, poach, and stew your food more regularly as these cooking methods create AGEs that are less harmful. If cooking at a high heat is required, cook at a lower temperature to minimize charring.

- **Eat less or keep clear of red meat:** Red meat includes items like lamb, hog, and beef. Even if it may be helpful if taken unprocessed, cooked at appropriate temperatures, and in moderation, red meat in general may have unfavorable health repercussions, most notably colon cancer. According to the WHO's International Agency for Research on Cancer (IARC), frequent intake of processed beef and red meat is probably carcinogenic. Why is eating red meat bad? To begin with, it may create considerable quantities of a molecule called trimethylamine N-oxide (TMAO) and high levels of TMAO have been connected with a range of disorders, such as cardiovascular difficulties and stomach and colon malignancies. Additional study is essential to completely comprehend TMAO's probable function in the development of illness.

Which diets are most wholesome?
If you want to live longer, why not learn from individuals who live in the "blue zones," which are places of the globe with the greatest life spans? Two of these "blue zones" are found in

the Mediterranean and Japan, where people adopt heart-healthy, nutrient-dense diets. They take in these things:

Mediterranean eating: This diet, which largely includes plant-based foods, is defined by a high consumption of vegetables, legumes, nuts, and olive oil as well as a minimal intake of processed foods, sweets, and meat. When coupled with food, red wine may be savored. The reason the Mediterranean diet is commonly referred to as the "Mediterranean plan" or lifestyle rather than a diet is that it differentiates from most others in that it doesn't exclude any foods; instead, it just restricts certain and emphasizes others.

Japanese diet: This plan focuses a premium on kelp and seaweed while urging a larger consumption of overall veggies and even less meat. Those who reside in Okinawa, Japan's blue zone, likewise eschew most fruits and legumes (with the exception of soybeans. Eating meals that are richer in nutrients may start you on the correct path to living a long, healthy life, even though there is no assurance that you won't fall ill.

CHAPTER FOUR

Heart concerns and heart health

As the biggest cause of mortality globally, cardiovascular disease is commonly referred to as the "silent pandemic." In just 2019 alone, it led to 18.6 million fatalities. Despite the worrisome data, the majority of premature deaths caused by atherosclerotic cardiovascular diseases (ASCVD) may be averted by adopting established, cost-effective therapies, such as improving awareness and eliminating modifiable risk factors.

Preventing Heart Disease

Usually, when we speak about prevention, we're talking about one of the three types: primordial, primary, or secondary prevention. All three have components in common, but they all start out differently and finish out differently.

A person at risk for heart disease should not have their first heart attack or stroke, require an angioplasty or other sort of surgery, or acquire any other kind of heart disease. This is the purpose of primary prevention. Primary prevention frequently focuses on patients who already have cardiovascular risk factors, such as high blood pressure or high cholesterol. Preventive care's major purpose is to decrease these risk factors via healthy lifestyle modifications and, if needed, medicines. Although endothelial dysfunction, atherosclerosis, and/or inflammation are already established and, for the most part, irreversible, the development of severe cardiovascular risk signs implies otherwise.

Secondary preventive therapies are initiated after a person suffers a heart attack or stroke, receives angioplasty or bypass surgery, or develops another sort of heart disease. It comprises stopping smoking, dropping weight if necessary, increasing exercise, and sticking to a healthy diet in addition to employing drugs like aspirin and/or statins to decrease cholesterol. Contrary to what the word would indicate, secondary prevention is not "closing the barn door after the horse has left." By following these actions, you may avoid early mortality, a second heart attack or stroke, and the start of heart disease. Second heart attacks, while they may seem evident, are the leading cause of mortality for people who survive a first attack.

The phrase "primordial" refers to anything that has always existed. Risk factors include high blood pressure, excessive cholesterol, excess weight, and finally cardiovascular events may be minimized by focusing on preventing the formation of inflammation, atherosclerosis, and endothelial dysfunction. The American Heart

Association today focuses major attention on primal prevention, a topic that was previously under-recognized, in its concept of perfect heart health and actions to assist individuals in reaching it. Primordial prevention is just what its name implies: the sooner you can start doing it, preferably from a young age, the more likely you are to be effective and protect yourself against heart disease.

Preventive measures for heart disease

By implementing the following five lifestyle alterations, your probability of accumulating cardiovascular risk factors and later getting heart disease may be greatly reduced:

Quitting Smoking: One of the finest things you can do for your health is to quit consuming cigarettes in any form. You might develop sluggish, get ill, and live less time as a consequence. Smoking is a tough habit to stop. Heart disease is one way it achieves this, among other others. In fact, across the course of a decades-long study involving more than 100,000 women, researchers evaluated the impact of smoking and quitting on mortality and found that roughly 64% of deaths among current smokers and 28% of deaths among former smokers were associated with cigarette smoking.

This research also proves that stopping smoking may substantially lessen a large portion of the danger that smoking raises. Furthermore, 20 years after quitting smoking, the higher risk for all-cause mortality, or dying from any cause, lowers to that of a "never-smoker". Nicotine, which is contained in tobacco products, is one of the most addictive compounds in the world. Smoking is one of the hardest harmful behaviors to quit because of this. Don't give up though; many smokers do stop! In fact, the number of former smokers in the US has overtaken that of current smokers.

Healthy weight: It's vital to maintain a healthy weight because being overweight and having a wide waistline are both related to heart disease and a number of other health concerns. In a research comprising more than a million women, the body mass index (BMI) was proven to be a considerable risk factor for coronary heart disease. The prevalence of coronary heart disease continuously rises with growing BMI. In the Nurses' Health Study and the Health Professionals Follow-Up Study, middle-aged women and men who gained 11 to 22 pounds after the age of 20 were up to three times more likely to develop heart disease, high blood pressure, type 2 diabetes, and gallstones than those who gained 5 pounds or less.

Those who put on more than 22 pounds had a considerably greater probability of getting these conditions. Weight and height have the reverse connection. The taller you are, the more you weigh. Because of this, scientists have established a range of measurements that account for both height and weight. BMI is the most widely utilized one. Your body mass index (BMI) may be computed by dividing your weight in kilograms by your height in square meters (kg/m2). Online BMI calculators and charts are also accessible. A healthy BMI is less than 25 kg/m2. Overweight is defined as a BMI of 25 kg/m2 to 29.9 kg/m2, and obesity is defined as a BMI exceeding 30 kg/m2. The waist's size is also crucial. Waist size, more so than BMI in persons who are not overweight, may be a marker of increased health risks. The National Institutes of Health formed an expert team to determine these helpful standards: Men should have a waist under 40 inches (102 cm), while women should have a waist under 35 inches (88 cm).

However, as we age, many of us become less active. Exercise and physical exercise are good strategies to avoid heart disease as well as many other illnesses and ailments.

Regular physical exercise: is one of the finest things you can do for your health. Heart disease, diabetes, stroke, high blood pressure, osteoporosis, and certain malignancies are less likely to arise as a consequence. Additionally, keeping a healthy weight, reducing stress, having better sleep, feeling happier, and enhancing cognitive function may all help older adults.

It's feasible to experience meaningful health benefits without partaking in marathon training. A brisk 30-minute walk five days a week will have great advantages for the majority of individuals. Any amount of exercise is more advantageous than none at all.

Exercise and physical activity are excellent for the body, while a sedentary lifestyle has the opposite consequence by boosting the chance of getting overweight and having a range of chronic ailments. According to studies, persons who lead less active lifestyles and spend more time each day sitting down, driving, or watching television are more likely to die early. Regardless of how much time was spent engaging in leisure-time physical activity, a 2013 research indicated that prolonged sitting was related to an enhanced risk of heart disease among women aged 50 to 79 who did not have cardiovascular disease at the start of the trial.

Eating healthily: Studies on the association between food and heart disease concentrated on particular vitamins and minerals as well as isolated substances like cholesterol and lipids. This research has been illuminating, but it has also brought us down some rabbit holes and reinforced incorrect beliefs about what a heart-healthy diet comprises. This is because humans consume food, not nutrition.

The best diet for heart disease prevention places an emphasis on fresh produce, whole grains, nuts, fish, poultry, and vegetable oils; it includes alcohol in moderation, if at all; and it restricts the consumption of red and processed meats, as well as refined carbohydrates, as well as foods and beverages with added sugar, sodium, and trans fats. The risks of stroke, diabetes, and heart disease were all cut by 20%, 33%, and 31%, respectively, among individuals who followed this eating pattern. A high intake of olive oil, nuts, fruits, vegetables, and cereals, a moderate consumption of fish and poultry, a low intake of dairy products, red meat, and processed meats, and a moderate intake of sweets and wine with meals are just a few of the qualities that characterize the Mediterranean diet. Each of these patterns stresses eating more whole grains, vegetables, fruits, legumes, and nuts while consuming less red and processed meat, as well as drinks with added sugar, while applying various scoring methodologies.

Two connected minerals, sodium and potassium, are necessary for maintaining a healthy heart and blood pressure. More potassium-rich meals and less salty food intake may dramatically lessen the risk of cardiovascular disease. Fruits, vegetables, legumes, low-fat dairy products, and many other foods contain potassium. However, consuming a lot of sodium-rich foods, such as processed bread, packaged snacks, canned products, and fast food meals, along with a low potassium diet may raise your risk of cardiovascular disease.

Increasing the amount and quality of sleep: Sleep deprivation has been linked to heart disease and may adversely influence other heart-related risk factors such as food, exercise, weight, blood pressure, and inflammation. Clinical sleep disorders, working late hours, poor sleep hygiene, and other factors may all lead to poor sleep. Speak with your doctor if you regularly have restless nights or do not feel rested during the day. It might assist in increasing sleeping patterns. Making and keeping a sleep routine, employing relaxation methods like stretching or meditation before night, exercising often, shutting off all electronic devices an hour before bedtime, and avoiding heavy meals, caffeine, and alcohol several hours before bed are a few examples.

Other things to consider
In addition to these five activities, the American Heart Association advocates decreasing cholesterol, blood sugar, and blood pressure as key variables for improving and sustaining cardiovascular health.

Keep a healthy blood pressure: You may maintain a healthy blood pressure level by eating a diet low in saturated fat, exercising regularly, and, if necessary, utilizing blood pressure medication. Your blood pressure should be maintained at about 140/90 mmHg. Try to check your blood pressure regularly whether you have high blood pressure, low blood pressure, or none of the two. You could discover abnormal blood pressure early and start treating it by doing this.

Keep your blood sugar under control: Diabetes raises your probability of acquiring CHD. You may regulate your blood sugar by maintaining a healthy weight, blood pressure, and degree of physical activity. Your blood pressure should be maintained under 130/80 mmHg.

You must take all drugs as recommended and at the right dose. Don't stop taking your medicine without first consulting a doctor as this can exacerbate your symptoms and put your health in danger.

Modification of enabling policies

It's crucial to bear in mind that unhealthy eating habits are influenced by
 a range of biological, social, economic, and psychological variables notwithstanding the effectiveness of adjusting one's own behavior. This is noted in a 2018 review article, which says "governments should focus on cardiovascular disease as a global threat and enact policies that will reach all levels of society and create a food environment wherein healthy foods are accessible, affordable, and desirable." The major picture in the paper (below) displays a number of government policies that may encourage healthy eating, such as enhancing nutrition labels, controlling food marketing, and supporting healthful learning and working situations.

CHAPTER FIVE

Managing the Runaway Cell

Almost every organ or tissue in the body may develop cancer, which is a wide category of disorders. These disorders are brought on by out-of-control, out-of-bounds aberrant cell proliferation that spreads to neighboring body parts and/or other organs. The penultimate stage, termed metastasizing, is a primary cause of cancer-related mortality. Neoplasm and malignant tumor are two more terminologies for cancer.

Cancer was the second biggest cause of mortality worldwide in 2018, accounting for an estimated 9.6 million deaths, or one in every six. Compared to women, who are more prone to acquire breast, colorectal, lung, cervical, and thyroid cancer, males are more likely to obtain lung, prostate, colorectal, stomach, and liver cancer.

Between 30% and 50% of cancer-related fatalities may be averted by modifying or eliminating important risk factors and putting into practice the currently indicated evidence-based preventative strategies. The burden of cancer might possibly be decreased via patient care and early cancer identification. The most cost-effective long-term method for controlling cancer is prevention.

To help prevent cancer, many significant risk factors may be addressed or avoided:

- Avoid using tobacco products like smokeless tobacco or cigarettes.
- Maintain a healthy weight.
- Eat a healthy, balanced diet with lots of fruits and vegetables.

- regular exercise Limit your alcohol consumption.
- Reduce occupational UV radiation exposure and avoid unneeded ionizing radiation exposure. Ensure safe and appropriate medical use of radiation in diagnosis and treatment.
- Avoid indoor smoking, indoor air pollution, and burning solid fuels in your dwelling.
- Receive regular medical care

Early cancer identification enhances the likelihood of survival while minimizing morbidity and treatment expenditures. Early cancer identification also enhances the probability that the illness may respond to effective treatment. Two distinct ways to enhance early detection:

- Early cancer detection finds instances of the ailment at its earliest stage. The objective of screening is to discover

people with anomalies indicative of a
particular disease or pre-cancer but who
have not yet developed any symptoms and
to send them right away for a diagnosis
and course of treatment.

- Treatment options include surgery, cancer
medicines, and/or radiation, either alone
or in combination. A multidisciplinary
team of cancer professionals suggests the
best course of action depending on the sort
of tumor, the stage of the illness, and other
criteria. The capabilities of the healthcare
system as well as the wishes of the
patients should be considered.

Palliative care, which aims to enhance the
quality of life for patients and their families, is a
crucial component of cancer treatment.
Survivorship care is a comprehensive strategy
for monitoring cancer recurrence and detecting
new malignancies, evaluating and treating the
long-term side effects of cancer and/or its

therapy, and providing resources to satisfy the needs of cancer survivors.

Immunotherapy, a sort of cancer treatment, helps your immune system fight cancer. The immune system in your body participates in the battle against diseases and infections. Its contents include organs, lymphatic system sections, and white blood cells.

Immunotherapy is a component of biological treatment. Biological therapy is a sort of cancer treatment that employs materials extracted from living creatures to attack the illness. The immune system recognizes aberrant cells, gets rid of them, and possibly slows or prevents the formation of many malignancies as part of regular function. For instance, immune cells may occasionally be detected in and around tumors. These cells, generally referred to as tumor-infiltrating lymphocytes, or TILs, are indications that the immune system has identified the tumor. TIL-positive cancer patients frequently had better outcomes than TIL-negative cancer patients.

Although the immune system may prevent or limit the spread of illness, cancer cells have methods of escaping the immune system. Cancer cells as an example:

- possess genetic changes that reduce the ability of their immune systems to recognize them.
- possess foreign proteins that hinder immune cells from functioning.
- The healthy cells in the region are modified in a manner that stops the immune system from fighting the cancer cells.

Cancer-fighting power of the immune system is boosted by immunotherapy.

CHAPTER SIX

Keeping a Healthy Weight as You Age

Obesity is a complex, chronic illness that may lead to increased body fat and, sometimes, poor health. Of course, having body fat alone is not a disease. However, having too much extra body fat might change the way your body functions. These modest modifications might deteriorate with time and have an adverse effect on one's health.

It is influenced by a wide range of factors, including genetic, behavioral, lifestyle, and environmental ones. Nearly every aspect of health is adversely impacted by obesity, including social interactions, respiration, mood, and sexual function. Additionally, it reduces lifespan and raises the likelihood of developing chronic illnesses like diabetes and cardiovascular disease.

Is obesity a condition that is weight-based?
Healthcare practitioners often use the Body Mass Index (BMI) to classify obesity in the general population. The average body weight to average height is calculated using the BMI. Obesity is often defined by healthcare experts as having a BMI of 30 or above. Although BMI has its limitations, it is a straightforward measurement that might make you aware of the health risks linked to obesity. Limitations include those with higher BMIs who have low levels of body fat, such as bodybuilders and athletes, who have more muscle mass. Obesity is another possibility when you are a "normal" weight. If your body weight is average but your body fat percentage is high, you can be at the same risk for health issues as someone with a higher BMI.

Medical practitioners have also observed racial differences in the maximum amount of extra weight that people may carry before it endangers their health. Black people are more likely than Asian people to have health risks at higher BMIs, while Asian people are more likely to experience health issues at lower BMIs.

Divide the result by the height in inches to get the BMI by multiplying the weight in pounds by 703. alternatively, multiply the height in meters squared by the weight in kg. Numerous internet calculators may be used to determine BMI.

What effects does obesity have on the body?
Obesity has a lot of effects on your body. Some of these negative effects of excess body fat are just mechanical. For instance, it is simple to tell the difference between carrying greater weight and putting more pressure on your bones and joints. Blood chemistry changes that increase your risk for diabetes, heart disease, and stroke are more subtle effects.

Metabolic modifications

Your body changes calories via your metabolism,your body's internal operations into energy. When there are more calories than you can ingest, your body converts the extra calories into lipids and stores them as body fat. When there is no longer any tissue for lipid storage, fat cells grow larger on their own. Expanded fat cells produce hormones and other inflammatory-causing chemicals. There are several effects of chronic inflammation on health. Among other things, it affects your metabolism by increasing insulin resistance. This shows that insulin is no longer an efficient way for your body to lower blood sugar and blood lipid levels (sugars and fats in your blood). Blood lipids (cholesterol and triglycerides) and blood sugar are both contributing factors to high blood pressure. When all of these risk factors are considered, the phrase "metabolic syndrome" is used. They are all included since they often complement one another. Furthermore, they promote further weight gain and make it more challenging to lose weight and sustain weight loss. The metabolic syndrome often contributes to obesity and the wide range of illnesses that are linked to it, including:

Type 2 diabetes: Depending on the gender allocated at birth, obesity specifically raises the risk of Type 2 diabetes by seven or twelve times, respectively. The risk increases by 20% for each additional BMI point. Additionally, when you lose weight, it becomes smaller.

Cardiovascular diseases: High blood pressure, high cholesterol, excessive blood sugar, or inflammation may all lead to cardiovascular problems such as coronary artery disease, congestive heart failure, heart attack, and stroke. An increase in these risks is correlated with your BMI. Cardiovascular disease is the leading cause of preventable death both worldwide and in the United States.

Excess fats: Extra fats in the blood go to the liver, which filters the blood and can cause fatty liver disease. When your liver begins to retain too much fat, it may result in chronic liver inflammation (hepatitis) and long-term liver damage (cirrhosis).

Direct outcomes

Excess body fat may suffocate the respiratory system's organs and put strain and stress on your musculoskeletal system. It supports:

- Asthma.
- Sleep apnea.
- the obese hypoventilation syndrome.
- Osteoarthritis.
- back pain.

According to the U.S. One in three obese people also suffer from arthritis, according to the Centers for Disease Control and Prevention. Studies show that for every 5 kg you gain, your risk of having knee arthritis increases by 36%. The good news is that a 10% weight loss together with exercise may significantly reduce arthritis pain and improve your quality of life.

Indirect outcomes:

Furthermore, obesity has indirect connections to:

- memory and cognitive abilities, including a higher risk of dementia and Alzheimer's disease.
- female infertility and complications throughout pregnancy.
- concerns with mental health and depression.
- Only a few instances are esophageal, pancreatic, colorectal, breast, uterine, and ovarian cancers.
- risk factors

Numerous underlying causes and aggravating conditions that contribute to obesity:

Genetics: The genes you acquired from your parents may have an impact on the amount and distribution of body fat you accumulate. In addition, your genes may have an impact on how well your body uses food as fuel, regulates your appetite, and burns calories as you exercise.

Obesity often runs in families. That isn't only due to the fact that they share DNA. Families often follow the same eating and exercise patterns.

Choice of lifestyle: A bad diet. Diets heavy in calories, lacking in fruits and vegetables, plentiful in fast food, and filled with high-calorie beverages and excessive portions all contribute to weight gain.

Calories: People have the capacity to eat a lot of calories.

You feel full from calories, especially those from alcohol. Aside from sugary soft drinks, other calorie-dense beverages also contribute to weight gain.

Inactivity: It's easier to eat more calories per day if you lead a sedentary lifestyle than you burn off via exercise and other daily activities. Staring at a computer, tablet, or phone screen qualifies as inactivity. There is a clear connection between screen usage and weight increase.

Specific conditions and remedies: Certain medical conditions, including hypothyroidism, Cushing syndrome, Prader-Willi syndrome, and others, may be associated with obesity in certain people. Medical conditions like arthritis, which may also lead to weight increase, may result in less activity.

Several drugs may result in weight loss if you don't make up for it with diet and activity. Beta-blockers, certain antidepressants, anti-seizure meds, diabetic medications, and antipsychotics are some of these drugs.

Age: Obesity may affect anybody, particularly young children. However, as you get older, hormonal changes and a less active lifestyle increase your chance of being obese. Your body's muscle mass starts to diminish as you get older. Muscle mass loss is often followed by a decline in metabolism. Additionally, these changes reduce calorie needs and can make it harder to lose weight. If you don't watch what you eat and increase your physical activity as you get older, you're more likely to gain weight.

The potential causes of an increase in calorie intake

Easy and fast to prepare meals: In neighborhoods and families where highly processed fast food and convenience foods are the norm, it's easy to consume a lot of calories. Given that these meals are high in sugar and fat and low in fiber and other nutrients, they may make you feel more hungry. Their elements promote obsessive eating patterns. In certain places, these may be the only readily available meal options due to cost and accessibility. 40% of American households, according to the Centers for Disease Control, are more than a mile distant from a healthy food store.

All things include sugar: The food industry is not primarily concerned with the maintenance of our health. It aims to promote products that we will become reliant on and want to buy more of. The top items on the list are sweets and sugary drinks, which are high in calories and low in nutritious value. However, a lot of sugar is added to everyday foods to increase their flavor and addictive potential. It is so pervasive that it has changed our expectations for taste.

Marketing and advertising: The products that we need the least but that the market forces us to buy the most are processed foods, sweets, and sugary drinks, all of which get heavy commercial promotion. Advertising portrays these products as everyday necessities that are part of daily life. Advertising plays a large part in the sale of alcohol and provides a lot of empty calories.

Psychological factors: Today's environment makes it common for boredom, loneliness, anxiety, and depression, all of which may lead to overeating. They could persuade us to eat more of certain high-calorie foods that activate our brain's pleasure centers. Humans have a natural need to eat when they're feeling down. **Our signals for hunger and fullness are regulated by hormones:** These regulatory activities may be compromised by a variety of conditions, including typical ones like stress and sleep deprivation as well as rare ones like genetic variations. Hormones may cause you to want food even when you don't need any additional calories. They could make it challenging for you to identify your point of weariness.

There are several factors that might lower the number of calories we burn:
Media addiction: As more of our jobs, purchases, and social interactions take place online, we spend more time on our phones and laptops. Thanks to streaming media and binge-watching, extended periods of inactive leisure are becoming more and more frequent.

Workforce modifications: Due to industrial changes that favor automation and computers, more people work at desks than on their feet nowadays. They also work longer hours.

Fatigue: The repercussions of sedentary behavior. According to research, being still for a long time makes you tired and unmotivated. Sitting makes the body stiffer and results in aches and pains that restrict movement. Additionally, it adds to general stress, which makes people feel exhausted.

planned neighborhoods. Many people lack access to surrounding venues to be active due to accessibility issues or safety worries. Most American houses are located more than half a mile from a park. They may not live in a walking location, and they might not see neighbors going about their everyday lives. When there is no alternative option for transportation, the bulk of people are forced to utilize their own automobiles.

Child care trends: Nowadays, kids don't spend as much time playing outside as they formerly did. They spend more time in enclosed childcare facilities, where there may not be adequate space or exercise equipment. This is partly a product of social trends that hold that children shouldn't play alone outside. Public spaces and inadequate access to top-notch childcare are other influencing variables. Free play often takes the place of viewing television in childcare settings.

Disability: Obesity is more prevalent in adults and children who have physical and learning challenges. Physical limitations, a lack of finances, and specialized education might all be factors.

How are overweight people handled and cared for?

Your overall health will establish your particular health profile.

treatment strategy. Before moving on to a longer-term weight loss plan, your medical expert will start by treating your most urgent health concerns. Sometimes they may advise making quick, immediate changes, like switching your prescription. The therapeutic process as a whole will be slower and probably include multiple factors. Studies have repeatedly shown that intensive, team-based programs with frequent, one-on-one interaction between you and your doctor are the most efficient ways to help people lose weight and keep it off.

Your treatment plan can include:

Diet adjustments: You alone will be able to determine the nutritional changes you need to make in order to lose weight. Some people could benefit from reducing their portion sizes or between-meal snacking. Some people may care more about changing what they eat than how much. Vegetable consumption is beneficial for practically everyone. Legumes, whole grains, fruits, and vegetables often contain more fiber and micronutrients than fat. Because they are higher in nutrients, less calories may make you feel fuller and happier.

Increased activity/exercise: Everyone is aware that in order to lose weight and maintain weight, both diet and exercise are necessary. However, a gym membership is not necessarily necessary to exercise. Simply walking at a reasonable pace is one of the best exercises for weight loss. Healthcare doctors recommend exercising about 30 minutes a day, five days a week. Regular walks before or after work, at lunch, or at other times might definitely help.

Psychological counseling: Counseling, support groups, and weight loss methods like cognitive behavioral therapy may be of use to you. Using these methods, your brain may be rewired to promote positive changes. They could also help you manage your stress and take care of any emotional or psychological problems that might be impeding your development. Having support on both a psychological and practical level may be helpful since our weight and efforts to reduce it affect us on many different levels.

Medication: Your doctor could advise using some medications in addition to other treatments. Although they don't provide a perfect answer, drugs may help you see weight loss from a new angle. For instance, some of the brain circuits that regulate your hunger may be blocked by drugs that reduce your appetite. For some people, this may just be a little piece of the puzzle, but it could be a bigger one.

How can I prevent gaining weight?
Obesity prevention is easier than obesity treatment after it has taken hold. Despite your aspirations to lose weight, your body attempts to control your hunger signals and energy expenditure in order to maintain the same body mass. You may want to act sooner rather than later to intervene if you've detected a trend of

recent weight increase in yourself or your kid, or if you have a family history of obesity. You may achieve your weight-loss objectives by looking at your behaviors and changing them. Two double-stuffed Oreos or a snack-size bag of potato chips are equal to 150 additional calories every day, which may add up to 10 more pounds in a year.

As an alternative, consider what you might do to burn an extra 150 calories each day, such as go on a hike, work out on an elliptical machine for 25 minutes, or walk the dog briskly for 35 minutes.

Instead of causing your blood sugar to spike and fall as processed snacks and candies do, whole foods are richer in fiber and lower the glycemic index. Healthy Diet: Fill your refrigerator with healthy meals, and save desserts and other delights for special occasions when you go out. Reduce screen time, go for a walk outside, learn to manage stress, and make an effort to get adequate sleep to keep hormone levels under control to ensure general wellness. Focus on making good changes and engaging in healthy activities rather than how your choices affect your weight.

Obesity's Effects on Life Expectancy

In spite of relatively steady obesity rates in the 1960s and 1970s, since the 1980s, two-thirds of American adults now qualify as overweight or obese. The obesity pandemic may result in a decrease in life expectancy in the United States in the twenty-first century, according to some experts' theories.

Obesity impairs almost every area of health, including reproductive, respiratory, cognitive, and emotional functions. It does this via a number of different channels, some as straightforward as the mechanical strain of bearing greater weight and others requiring subtle adjustments to hormones and metabolism. Diabetes, heart disease, and certain types of cancer are just a few of the dangerous conditions that obesity makes more likely.

The bottom line

Nearly every aspect of health is adversely impacted by obesity, including social interactions, respiration, mood, and sexual function. Additionally, it reduces lifespan and raises the likelihood of developing chronic illnesses like diabetes and cardiovascular disease. It's not usually a lifetime issue to be obese. Through food, exercise, medication, and even surgery, a person may reduce weight. But losing weight is far more difficult than gaining it. Preventing obesity at an early age and continuing throughout one's career has the potential to improve both public and individual health, alleviate suffering, and save yearly healthcare costs by billions of dollars. If you are fat, you run the risk of experiencing some major health problems. That does not mean you already satisfy those standards. Additionally, it does not indicate that you have no choices for handling them. The risks are real, but they may be handled or avoided. To minimize them, your doctor would suggest you lose weight. Even though it will be challenging, it is still feasible.

CHAPTER SEVEN

How to Maintain Strength and Stability as You Age

Growing emphasis is being given to aging in general and effective aging in particular by the scientific community. Numerous initiatives aimed at improving the physical and mental health of the elderly have been launched. People are more susceptible to falling because of age-related losses in physical performance and cognitive abilities, which result in a loss of balance, coordination, and muscular strength. Human balance is the ability to adapt to environmental disturbances by maintaining a position (such as sitting or standing), changing postures, and avoiding falling. It is a complex, multifaceted phrase related to postural control.

In addition to the danger of fractures associated with falls, balance is one of the essential elements of many daily activities, both professional and recreational; as a result, a reduction in this ability may have a detrimental influence on the quality of life. A specific definition of the word "fall" has been proposed as follows: "accidentally coming to rest on the ground, floor, or other lower level, excluding intentional change of position to rest in furniture, wall, or other objects." A "recurrent faller" is a person who falls twice in the course of six months, which happens to one in three older citizens annually.

Elderly falls, which account for 40% of all injury-related deaths in this population, are alarming occurrences that can lead to fractures, long-term disability, chronic pain, and loss of independence. They also have significant social and public health repercussions that necessitate expensive long-term treatments. The severity of injuries caused by falls varies significantly, from minor scrapes and bruises to major fractures and, in a few rare cases, fatal traumas. Patients with osteoporosis are more likely to sustain femoral fractures or vertebral body fractures, especially if they fall on stairs or hard surfaces. Inactivity, which is known to cause age-related decline in biological function, may lead to physical impairment. To the extent that the adage "exercise is medicine" has been used, exercise does have a significant role in avoiding a variety of age-related disorders, including cancer, metabolic, cardiovascular, and bone quality deterioration.

Numerous studies have shown that physical exercise reduces the risk of falling in older citizens, improves balance, and stops muscle wasting. Leg strength training is particularly helpful in preventing falls since lower-limb weakness has been shown to be a significant risk factor for falling. Indicators of postural control in particular may be used to assess the risk of falling.

Furthermore, current research has examined balancing training as a substantial intervention to lessen the physiological loss of balance control in the elderly and has shown that it is an effective way to improve balance and postural control. Stiffness and reduced joint range of motion, sarcopenia and lost muscular strength, cognitive decline, and adaptations to the sensory systems, such as worsened vision and hearing, are age-related changes to the body's capacity for balance.

Why the risk of falling rises with age

The aging process has an effect on the tissues and systems of every individual. Although each person's rate and degree of aging may differ, physical degeneration is a normal part of becoming older. The majority of people think that aging starts in their 60s, but in truth, we spend the majority of our lives in a condition of decline, which often begins in our 30s.

The following are a few common reasons why older persons fall:

- First of all, as we age, our muscles naturally lose flexibility and strength, making it more difficult to maintain balance and stability. Poor balance and a lack of strength are two of the main causes of falls.
- Second, chronic conditions like diabetes, Parkinson's disease, or arthritis are often present in elderly people and may make them less stable, coordinated, and mobile in general.
- Furthermore, a number of commonly used therapies by elderly people, such as sedatives or blood pressure drugs, may make them sleepy or cause a drop in blood pressure, which raises their risk of falling.
- The visual changes brought on by aging, such as diminished depth perception, decreased peripheral vision, and difficulty

differentiating colors or contrasts, may
make it harder to navigate and notice
threats. Environmental risks include
crowded paths, loose rugs or carpets,
slippery floors, and uneven surfaces may
significantly increase the risk of falls in
older people.
- Other problems elderly people may have
who lead sedentary lives or do little
physical activity include reduced strength,
flexibility, and balance.

Avoiding falls

The negative impacts of aging, such as falls and
accidents, may be reduced by making changes
to one's lifestyle, such as engaging in regular,
long-term exercise. Older people may reduce
their risk of falling by keeping their homes safe,
managing chronic illnesses, discussing
medications with medical experts, eating a
healthy diet, and getting regular eye
examinations.

Physical therapists use a range of exercises to improve their patients' balance. But it's important to keep in mind that everyone should see a doctor or a physical therapist before starting any fitness program to determine the exercises that are most suited to their unique needs. I often suggest to my patients that they do the five forms of exercise listed below to improve their balance:

Coordination and proprioception, the body's awareness of its location in space, may benefit from balance exercises. By putting the nervous system through balance-testing drills like heel-toe walking and standing on one leg, the nervous system becomes better at coordinating movement and maintaining balance. According to a thorough research study that examined over 8,000 senior citizens, balance and functional activities reduce the incidence of falls by 24%.

Lifting weights and using resistance bands are two exercises that develop physical strength and power. Strengthening the muscles in the legs, hips, and core may assist older people in maintaining their balance and stability. Our research suggests that strength training may also speed up walking and reduce the risk of falling. The focus of the peaceful martial art of tai chi is on weight-shifting and slow, controlled movements. According to study, it could improve the balance, strength, and flexibility of senior people. Numerous pooled studies have shown a 20% reduction in the likelihood of falls when tai chi is practiced.

Certain yoga techniques may help with balance and stability. The tree position, the warrior stance, and the mountain pose are three different postures that might improve balance. Yoga is best performed while being instructed by a qualified instructor who can adjust the poses to each student's level of fitness.

During flexibility training, stretching the muscles and joints may broaden the range of motion and reduce stiffness. Increasing the range of motion may make it safer for seniors to walk and reduce the risk of falls brought on by mobility problems.

Using assistive technology may be helpful when there are problems with strength or balance. Studies examining the use of canes and walkers by elderly people have shown that these aids can improve balance and mobility. Learning how to utilize assistive technology correctly from a physical or occupational therapist may boost safety.

To find out more about the risk of falling, you should also:

- See a healthcare expert.
- Discuss the side effects of prescription medications often with a doctor or pharmacist to understand them.

- Have your hearing and vision checked annually.
- Seek the help of your friends, family, and companions.
- Any adjustments to your medication regimen should be discussed with your doctor.
- Inform your doctor if you fall.
- Ask a friend or a family member to inspect your home for trip hazards.
-

Progress may be made at any moment toward improving balance and lowering risk factors. Also remember that fall prevention may increase freedom, reduce financial load and danger of injuries, and potentially save lives.

CHAPTER EIGHT

Sleep as a Medicine for Aging

Although it may seem strange, when you sleep, your body is really busy. A multitude of mechanisms help your brain, cardiovascular system, and other organs work as best they can.

Because of this, obtaining adequate sleep may improve your overall health and prolong your life. Both little sleep and enough sleep may have the opposite effect. Finding the sweet spot when you're getting the ideal amount of sleep for your body might help you live a long and healthy life. In terms of the amount recommended for their age group, teenagers and younger children often need more sleep than adults do.

Sleeping less than seven hours a night on a regular basis may be detrimental to your cardiovascular, endocrine, immune, and neurological systems, according to a study. Potential adverse effects of sleep deprivation include obesity, diabetes, heart disease, hypertension, anxiety, depression, alcohol abuse, stroke, and an increased risk of different malignancies.

Why Your Body Needs Sleep
In addition to helping you feel more refreshed, sleep helps your muscles, organs, and brain cells repair and replenish each night. Sleep controls both your metabolism and the release of hormones. When these systems are out of balance as a consequence of sleep loss, your chance of developing health problems may increase.

Sleeping less than seven hours a night on a regular basis may be detrimental to your cardiovascular, endocrine, immune, and neurological systems, according to a study. Potential adverse effects of sleep deprivation include obesity, diabetes, heart disease, hypertension, anxiety, depression, alcohol abuse, stroke, and an increased risk of different malignancies. Even though having too little sleep may increase your risk on its own, it's also possible that a more serious issue is preventing you from obtaining enough rest. For instance, sleep deprivation has been linked to obesity and heart disease. However, it's also likely that obesity and heart disease already present are contributing to breathing problems like sleep apnea, which are hurting your sleep and, as a result, your overall health and longevity.

If you don't get enough sleep, your chances of being involved in potentially fatal situations increase. A 2014 study found that obtaining seven to eight hours of sleep each night lowers your risk of being in a car accident by 33%. According to the research, those who receive less sleep at night may be to blame for 9% of all road accidents.

Effects of Too Much Sleep on Health

Dangerous is not just getting enough sleep. Additionally, excessive napping might be a sign of health problems. One study found no relationship between the other chronic medical conditions connected to poor sleep and extended sleep, which is defined as more than 10 hours each night. Another study with almost 30,000 individuals found that those who slept nine hours or more each night had a 23% greater risk of stroke than people who slept seven to eight hours each night. Those who slept for more than nine hours or more often than 90 minutes throughout the day had a stroke risk that was 85% greater.

Consistently needing more sleep than normal might be a sign that something is wrong. Excessive sleepiness may be caused by a range of factors, such as sleep disorders or sleep apnea, which can all contribute to poor overall sleep quality. If this is the case, you should see a doctor to have your sleeping habits examined. Depression may also cause a person to sleep excessively (or insufficiently, or get up too early). It's critical to bring up this issue with a medical professional when less overt depressive symptoms appear.

How Much Sleep Promotes Longevity?

The recommended amount of sleep each night is between seven and eight hours, according to studies. However, the amount of sleep that each individual needs varies.

In one study, almost 21,000 twins were followed by researchers for more than 22 years. They inquired about the twins' sleeping habits and tracked the twins' development. The majority of twins grow raised in the same setting and have similar genetic make-ups, making them good research subjects. As a consequence, scientists are able to identify how a behavior—such as how much sleep someone gets—affects a result.

The participants were questioned at the beginning and end of the study. The questions focused on the amount, effectiveness, and use of sleep aids. The likelihood of death was greater for those who slept less than seven hours or more than eight hours each night (24% and 17%, respectively), according to the research. When sleep medications were taken, the chance of mortality increased by around a third, indicating a problem falling asleep.

Suggestions for a Better Night's Sleep
If you don't currently get enough sleep, you may take the following steps to improve your sleep:
Keep your bedtime and waking time consistent, even on the weekends.
Device use should be avoided just before bed, and at night, keep them out of your bedroom.

As dark as you can make your bedroom.
Avoid consuming coffee, eating, or drinking
anything before night.
a regular movement.

Here are some suggestions to help you get more rest, both in terms of amount and quality:

- Maintain a consistent sleep schedule; inconsistent patterns may cause sleep problems. Consider establishing a consistent wake-up and bedtime for every day, including on the weekends or on days off.
- Even though you may like scrolling through social media in bed, studies have shown that utilizing devices for at least 30 minutes before bed might result in bad sleep. If you feel this is a contributing reason to your sleep troubles, you can

think about implementing a "no device in the bedroom" policy to see if it helps.

- Limit your intake of coffee, alcohol, and heavy meals just before bed. Later in the sleep cycle, alcohol may disrupt sleep patterns. Large meals eaten too soon to bedtime may make it difficult for you to fall asleep since they promote digestion when your body is trying to sleep.

- By making it simpler for you to do so during the day, exercise may aid in helping you achieve a decent night's sleep. However, timing your workouts might be crucial. If you generally have greater energy after working out, doing out too close to bedtime can keep you up all night. Generally speaking, you should give yourself two hours between the end of your workout and bedtime.

- Change your sleeping arrangement: If you're having difficulties falling asleep, trying a comfy couch or a different bed can help. Some individuals discover that all it takes to fall asleep is a fresh start someplace else.

- Write down your thoughts and keep them out of your mind: Due to continuous anxiety, some people may have trouble falling asleep. If you experience this, consider having a notepad next to your bed so that you may jot down any thoughts that come to you. Writing down your thoughts for the next day might aid in your relaxation if you feel the need to remember them.

- Create the ideal sleeping environment: You may want to consider lowering the temperature in your bedroom, removing any glaring lights, or using a fan or noise machine to block out outside sounds since the environment you sleep in may alter the duration and quality of your sleep.

CHAPTER NINE

The Cost of Ignoring Emotional Health

If you shattered your leg, would you still disregard it? You probably wouldn't. You'd go to the hospital as fast as you could to have it taken care of before it became worse. Exactly the same holds true for your mental health. If you see a change in your mental health, it's critical to get help. Numerous psychological conditions might make it difficult for you to maintain relationships, enjoy life, or take care of everyday tasks. Taking care of your mental health is an essential component of healthy aging.

Mental illnesses are medical conditions that have an impact on a person's thinking, feelings, mood, interpersonal interactions, and daily functioning. Similar to how diabetes is a pancreatic disease, mental illnesses are medical issues that often lead to a diminished capacity to manage the demands of everyday life. Serious mental health conditions include significant depression, schizophrenia, bipolar disorder, obsessive compulsive disorder (OCD), anxiety disorders, post-traumatic stress disorder (PTSD), and borderline personality disorder. The good news is that people with mental health issues may recover.

Mental illnesses may have an effect on people of any age, race, religion, or financial status. Character faults, a poor upbringing, or a lack of personal strength do not cause mental illnesses. Although they may be addressed, mental health problems cannot be overcome via willpower and have no bearing on a person's moral character or intelligence. Most people who have been diagnosed with a serious mental illness are able to regulate their symptoms by actively participating in a unique treatment plan.

In addition to prescription medication, psychosocial therapies, including cognitive behavioral therapy, interpersonal counseling, peer support groups, and other community services, may be part of a treatment plan and aid in recovery. In terms of overall health and wellness, including the recovery from mental illness, transportation, food, exercise, sleep, friends, and worthwhile paid or volunteer activities all play a part.

Mental illness often strikes while a person is in their prime, in their teens or early 20s. Although people of all ages are in danger, the young and the old are especially vulnerable. Without treatment, mental illness has terrible consequences for both the individual who is afflicted and society at large. Disorders of the mind that are not addressed may result in poor quality of life, unnecessary disabilities, unemployment, drug abuse, homelessness, and unjust incarceration. Untreated mental illness damages the American economy by more than $100 billion annually.

The most effective treatments for serious mental illnesses nowadays are highly successful; between 70% and 90% of patients see a significant reduction in symptoms and an improvement in quality of life. These treatments include pharmacological and psychosocial therapy and support. With the aid of appropriate, effective medicine and a wide range of therapies suited to their needs, the majority of people who live with serious mental illnesses may considerably minimize the consequences of their conditions and achieve a satisfying degree of accomplishment and independence. It's crucial to become proficient at making strategies to limit the progression of illness.

Early identification and treatment are essential, and by ensuring access to therapies and supports for recovery that have been shown to be beneficial, recovery is sped up and the potential for subsequent disease-related harm is reduced. Stigma undermines the idea that mental diseases are real, treatable medical conditions. Because of stigma and an unwarranted sense of powerlessness, barriers to effective treatment and rehabilitation have been allowed to increase in our society. These barriers include psychological, structural, and financial.

Conditions of the Ill Mind
- Changes in personality, conduct, or emotions ("lack of insight")
- utilizing alcohol or drugs a variety of physiological ailments that have unclear causes (including headaches, stomachaches, and broad "aches and pains") are used incorrectly.
- Suicidal thoughts, extreme fear of growing weight, inability to manage stress

and problems of everyday life, or anxiety about appearance.

- modifications to academic performance persistent worry or anxiety, such as skipping bedtime or going to school
- extreme activity and frequent nightmares
- persistent antagonism or disobedience, frequent rage attacks

There is always a chance of a crisis when a mental illness is present. Crisis episodes associated with mental illness may be quite frightening.

Alert Signs: Increased alcohol and drug use violent behavior separation from family, friends, and community
sudden mood swings, dangerous or reckless actions
Suicidal thoughts constitute an emergency in mental health. If you or a loved one starts to

engage in any of these actions, call 911 or get emergency medical help.

Buying a gun vs. gathering and storing narcotics

Make a contribution by finishing up open tasks, such as paying bills or organizing personal records

saying good-bye to family and friends

Risk Factors

46% of suicide victims had a confirmed mental health condition, according to studies.

Additional elements that might raise a person's risk of suicide include:

- drug addiction in the family and a history of suicide. Drugs may cause violent mood fluctuations in the mind that heighten suicidal thoughts.
- Intoxication. More than one-third of suicide fatalities are related to alcohol use.
- getting weapons a serious or persistent illness

- Gender. Despite the fact that more women than men attempt suicide, males are nearly 4 times more likely to die by suicide.
- a history of trauma or abuse
- persistent anxiety
- a recent calamity or loss

Taking action as soon as depressive signs are noticed

Your emotional and physical health are equally important. Studies indicate that depression is a significant problem among seniors, especially when there are physical limitations. It's OK to have occasional emotional lows. Try to speak about your feelings with a friend or family member to help you get through these moments. As you become older, you should be more conscious of your mental health and wellness since depression risk increases.

The Connection Between Emotional and Physical Health

Seniors who are mentally unwell are less likely to actively engage in physical fitness-promoting activities. When your emotions are in check, you'll be more motivated to focus on adopting lifestyle choices that will enhance your general health, including eating a balanced diet and working out. Your physical health may be severely harmed by anxiety and other mental health problems. Changes in appetite, sleepless nights, and physical pain are some symptoms of the problems. If you are exhibiting any of these symptoms, it is imperative that you get help at a senior healthcare facility to prevent them from further impairing your physical health.

An Aging Brain Can Be Rejuvenated by a Positive Attitude

Emotional optimism may improve cognitive performance and lower the risk of dementia, according to research. A positive outlook also serves as protection against more serious mental health problems like depression. Even though many people fear aging, it is a reality that we must all embrace. To age gracefully both mentally and physically, make sure to engage in activities where you feel like you have a purpose, be physically active, and be socially engaged. You will age more gracefully the more emotionally stable you are.

Additional Tips for a Long and Healthy Life

According to studies, a sense of meaning or purpose in life is connected to better sleep, a healthier weight, more physical activity, and reduced levels of inflammation in certain people. It also promotes optimism. Better health among older persons may enable them to contribute more to their families, communities, and society at large. This corresponds to the ability to work until retirement age, assist younger generations with childcare or other household duties, engage in fulfilling hobbies, and take part in civic activities. It also entails having more physical stamina and mobility. As a result, people have a sense of purpose and meaning.

Social connections - Studies on seniors (50 years and older) show that loneliness and social isolation are associated with a higher risk of disease, disability, and mortality. In the 11,302 older individuals who participated in the U.S. Health and Retirement study, over 20% met the criteria for loneliness. Chronic loneliness increased the risk of early death by 57% compared to never having experienced it, while social exclusion increased the risk by 28%. Participants who reported both loneliness and social isolation exhibited biological aging (for instance, chronic inflammation that increases the risk of morbidities). On the other hand, persons who are experiencing cognitive impairment could have less social interactions because they find it more difficult to initiate and maintain discussions.

Brain stimulation - Engaging in mentally demanding activities, such as learning a new skill, language, or fitness regimen during downtime, may reduce the risk of cognitive decline. A lower incidence of dementia, Alzheimer's disease, and cognitive impairment has been substantially related in studies to higher education and intellectually demanding jobs.

Animal studies have shown that calorie restriction over the course of a lifetime, such as intermittent fasting, may lengthen life. Fasting leads to improved blood glucose regulation, heightened resilience to stress, decreased inflammatory response, and reduced production of potentially damaging free radicals in the body. When you fast, your cells purge or repair damaged molecules. These effects could prevent the development of chronic illnesses including obesity, diabetes, cardiovascular disease, cancer, and brain degradation like Alzheimer's disease. The practice of intermittent fasting in animals also has additional advantages, such as better coordination, balance, and memory. Human studies have shown improved insulin sensitivity, lowered blood pressure, decreased LDL cholesterol, and weight loss. Randomized controlled studies and human research are still needed to fully understand how fasting affects aging and longevity.

www.ingramcontent.com/pod-product-compliance
Lightning Source LLC
Chambersburg PA
CBHW070811260726
48660CB00005B/1801